W9-CSG-897

Support the Girls

Support the Girls

Bra Art for Breast Health

Compiled by the
West Parry Sound
Health Centre Foundation

Second Story Press

NATIONAL LIBRARY OF CANADA CATALOGUING IN PUBLICATION DATA

Support the girls : bra art for breast health / compiled by
the West Parry Sound Health Centre Foundation.

ISBN 978-1-926920-73-3

1. Brassieres in art. 2. Art, Canadian—21st century.
3. Laughter—Therapeutic use--Anecdotes. 4. Breast—Cancer—
Patients—Ontario—Anecdotes. I. West Parry Sound Health
Centre Foundation

N8217.B68S96 2012   704.9'493914230971315   C2011-908657-3

Design by Melissa Kaita

Printed and bound in Canada

*Second Story Press gratefully acknowledges the support of the
Ontario Arts Council, the Ontario Media Development Corporation,
and the Canada Council for the Arts for our publishing program. We
acknowledge the financial support of the Government of Canada
through the Canada Book Fund.*

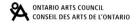 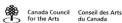

Published by
SECOND STORY PRESS
20 Maud Street, Suite 401
Toronto, ON
M5V 2M5
www.secondstorypress.ca

Foreword

Can a book about breast health be both beautiful and funny? This one is.

When the women from a small community needed to raise money to buy a mammography machine for the local hospital, it wasn't laughter that led them to the 'art-bra' project. It was the fear of breast cancer and the need for early detection that motivated them. But the results of their fundraising project are full of fun and whimsy. People from near and far responded to the call to craft an 'art-bra,' and send in their creations along with the stories behind them.

You will smile at the bras that have turned into works of art, with names such as Got Milk?, Lucky Charms, BRAhama Mama, Floss Your Teets, and Cradles of Civilization. The book showcases four dozen of the bras, with accompanying personal stories that celebrate the curative power of laughter. Even hockey great Bobby Orr was onside and signed one of the sportier examples.

The bras, pieces of art from the heart, come from breast cancer sufferers and survivors, healthcare workers, friends and family. These 'bra-artistas' will inspire you and move you to tears – both of laughter and sadness. Their fabulous creations and their stories bring a sense of lightness and hope to an all-too serious problem.

*Thanks to 2,459 donors (individuals and organizations)
the West Parry Sound Health Centre installed its
new digital mammography machine January 2012.*

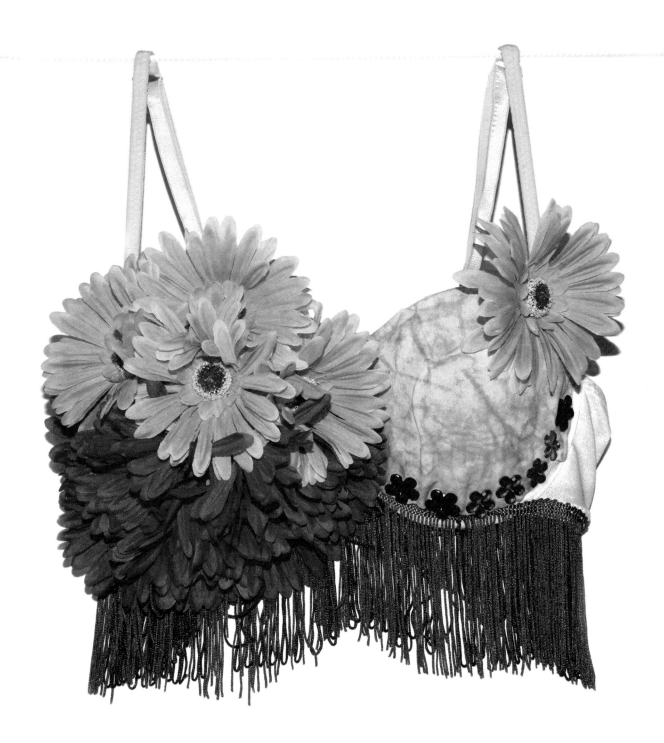

Mums Forever

My mother was the inspiration for this bra. She was a woman with many facets. She was a wife, a mother to five, a grandmother, a war veteran, and a career woman. Her three daughters were raised to know that the only limitations in your life are those you put on yourself. As an only child she always felt that she had missed something, so for her, it was definitely 'family first.' Even today, fifteen years after we lost her, our family meets at every holiday and celebrates her life and our lives. This bra commemorates the fun-loving "hippy" part of her character. We all miss her very much.

Diana DeLuca

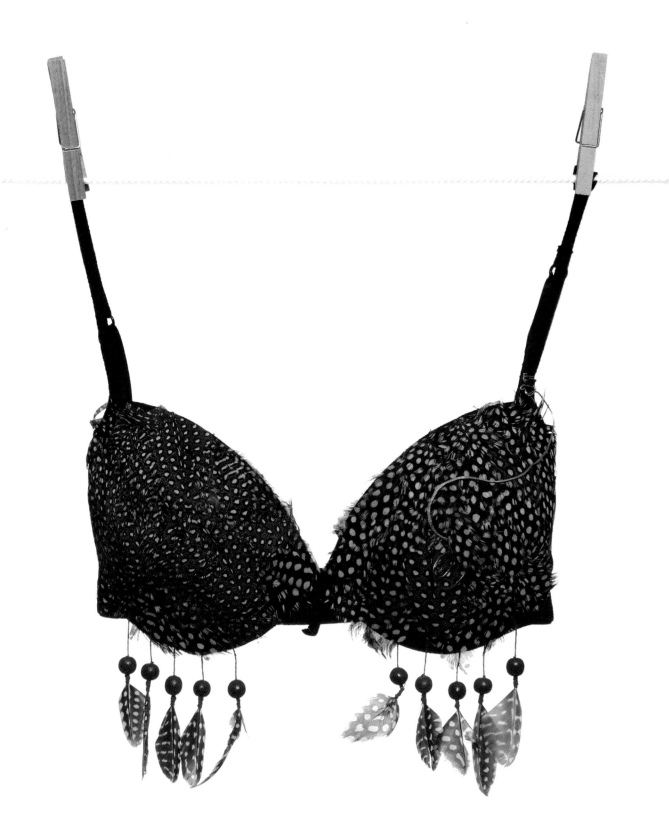

Fly High

Aboriginal peoples believe that the power of the world always works in circles, as demonstrated by the sun and the moon, the seasons, the nest of a bird, the life of a woman from childhood to childhood. In the old days all power came from the sacred hoop of the nation and so long as the hoop was unbroken the people flourished. In indigenous societies, coming together in a circle is as natural as sitting around a campfire. When we come together in a circle there is the power of many voices becoming one – a voice with experience from many perspectives is able to discover options and solutions that often go beyond what one person could generate.

The feather of the guineafowl, a bird of protection as well as a symbol of human effort to survive, adds to the power of the circle. With this strength, of the circle and the feather, we should always endeavor to fly high. After all, in Africa there is a belief that birds are the souls of human beings who have reached a high state of perfection.

Riley Harris

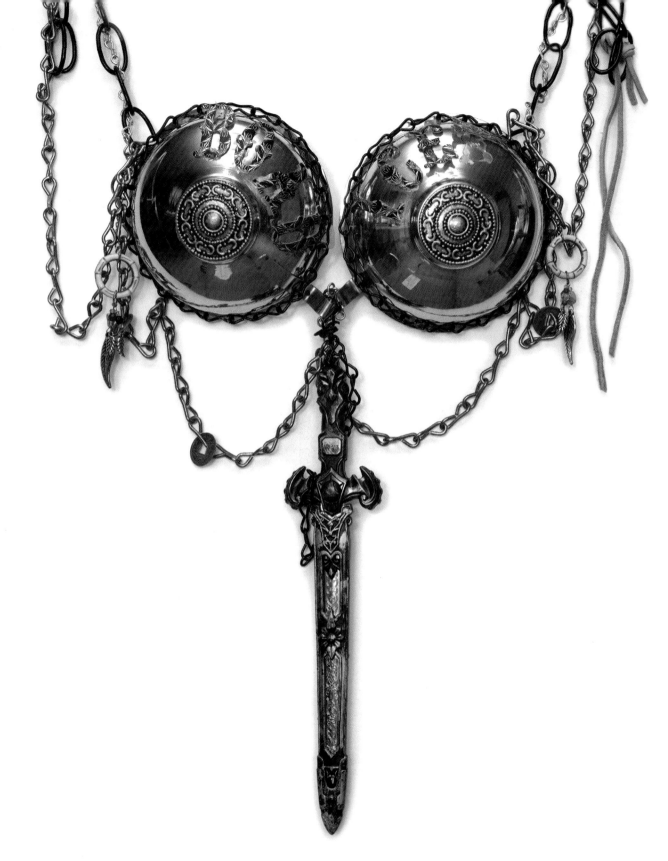

Stone-Age Bra

I am a male radiological technologist and I submitted this bra to bring awareness to the fact that males can also get breast cancer. Most men have no inkling that they can also get breast cancer, but we have positive mammograms on men, especially older men, who have similar symptoms to women's. A personal male friend recently succumbed to this cancer. Since cancer has been present from ancient times, the "Flintstone" era seemed an appropriate theme.

Tudor Randell

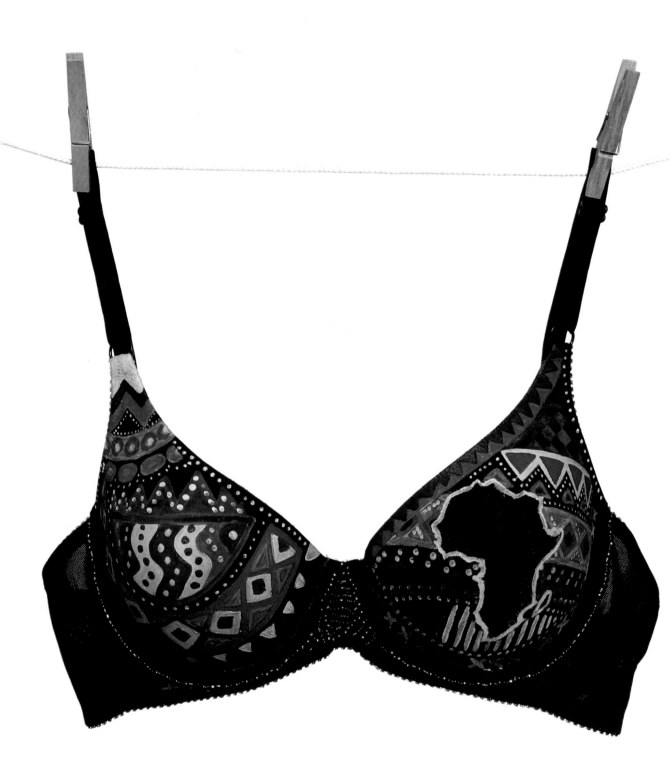

Cradles of Civilization

Africa is said to be the cradle of civilization. It is where humanity's story started and for that reason it is a symbol of life – life into which we are brought by our mothers and through which we are sustained by their care. Africa is where my mother was born and where I started my own story. To me it seems a mother to us all, and for this reason Africa is the perfect symbol to express my support of all mothers and daughters who are currently battling breast cancer. It also serves as a reminder that we are all connected and are fundamentally the same, and that if we realize we are more similar than different, we can solve many of the problems that face our world today, cancer included.

Jess Fargher

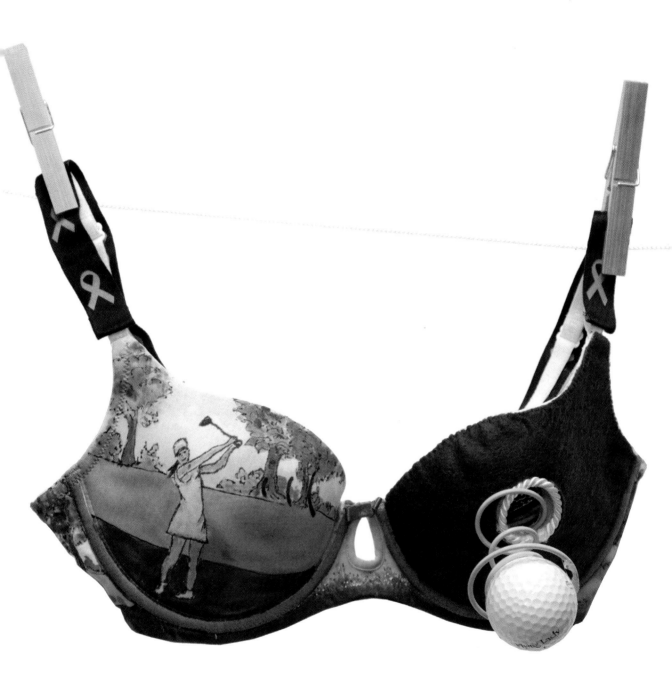

Hole in One

A hole in one…a hole in oneself…a hole in your heart.
The domino effects of breast cancer.
So many wounds, too many losses.
Physical, psychological.
Victims, family.

A gold heart is buried in the "hole" of this bra.
It is a healing heart.
With time. With faith.

If you are a golf pro, the odds of getting a hole in one are
one in 3,756.
The odds of a woman developing breast cancer in her
lifetime? One in nine.
Switching those odds – now that will be the time to celebrate!

Debbie Anderson and Paula Attwell

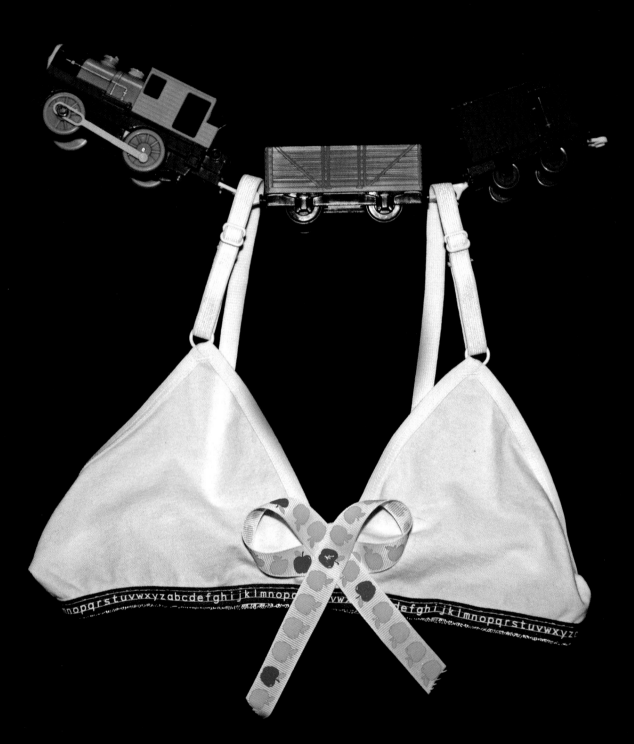

Training Bra

Three months before my thirty-second birthday I had a total hysterectomy. I had been diagnosed with endometriosis – and had a cyst the size of an orange, the doctor said. My husband and I were content to be childless until my absent biological clock reappeared at age forty-seven. Eighteen months later, I was climbing the steps of the Great Wall of China with my newly adopted one-year-old daughter in my arms.

This bra is for my now-budding twelve-year-old in a year when I am five times her age. What started as a playful pun on the concept of "training" made me think of learning. School is a huge part of a tween's life, so I added the school-themed bow and trim. Learning to be a woman – my daughter is a woman in training.

Maryann Madore

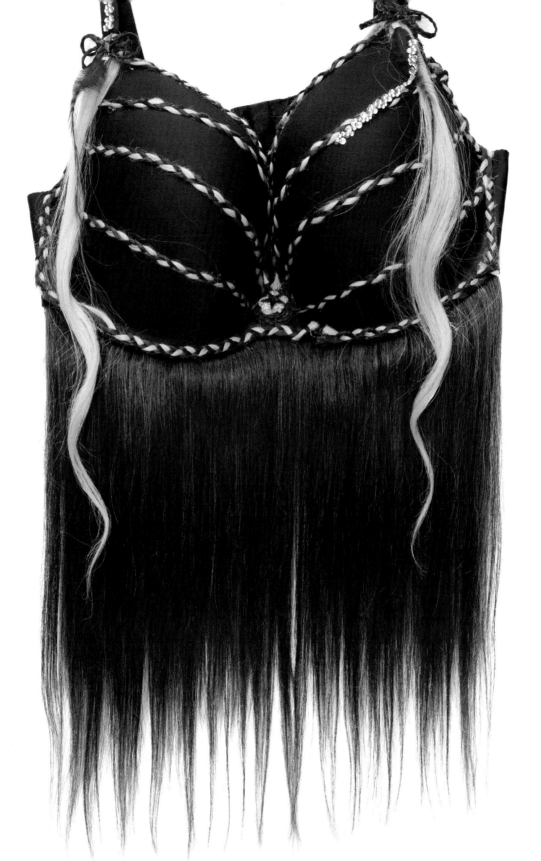

Savvy 'DDD' Lite

Hair is important. It makes you feel feminine. It can make or break your day. When your hair looks good, you feel good. The women of our salon and spa created Savvy DDD Lite using real human hair in our bra as a fitting tribute to women.

First we brainstormed, then, over the course of two weeks, we placed every hair on the DDD cups, adding just the right touch of glitter and decoration. With its brown, red, blonde, and black strands, the bra is unique and represents both women and the salon.

Participating in the project was a no-brainer for us. Some of our clients have had breast cancer and barely a day goes by that the topic isn't broached. The bra not only helped raise money, but also awareness. When Savvy DDD Lite was on display in the salon, it caught everyone's attention and became the jumping off point for many conversations. It also generated a few more donations for the cause.

Savvy Salon

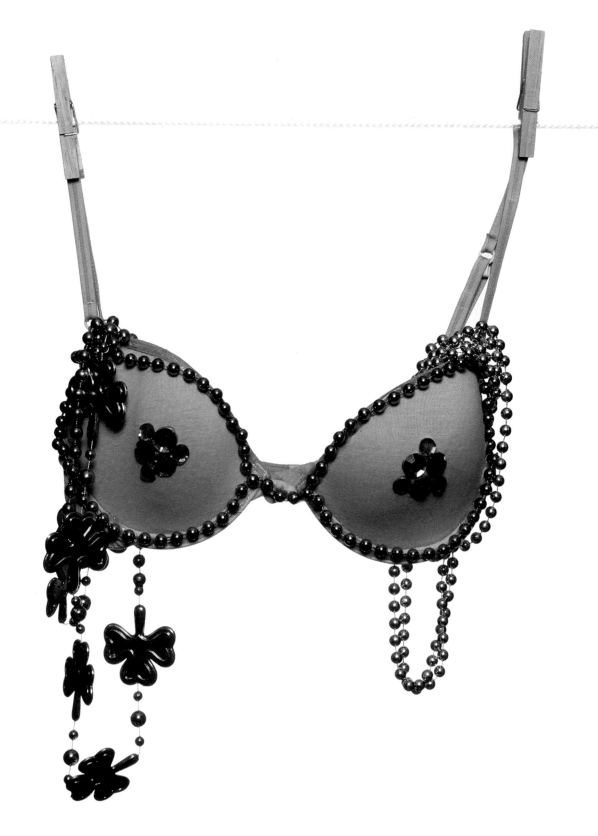

Lucky Charms

Cancer – many types – runs in our family. I have had melanoma, others have had to deal with basal cell and sarcoma skin cancer, leukemia, bowel, colon, and lung cancers.

Many of my friends have had breast cancer. After diagnosis, they all felt overwhelming fear for a short time, then gracefully dealt with what they had to do to get rid of it. Not all have succeeded in winning the race. These wonderful "sisters" have stayed with me through the years through my great memories and photos. But thank heavens I also have friends who have lived ten to fifteen years post diagnosis.

Lucky Charms was my first decorated bra. To create it, I rescued my daughter's first bra, which happened to be a charming green, from the recycling donation crate. Out came the pins, sequins, glue gun – what better way to cheer for a cure than designing a saucy, good-luck shamrock bra?

To all my wonderful friends, those here and those who have passed on: "May the road rise to meet you. May the wind be always at your back."

Helen Ayers

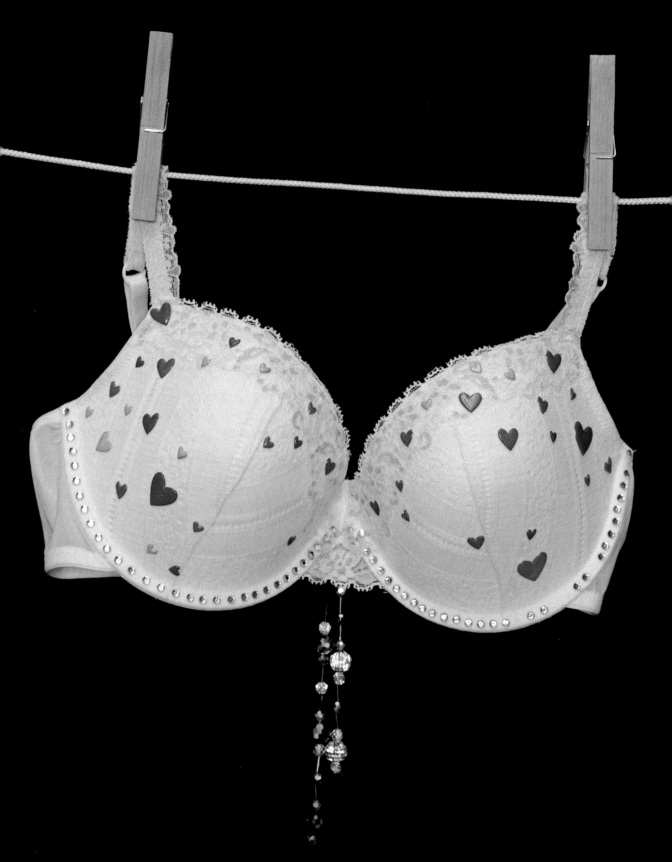

Friends Forever

In 1975, my friend Roseanne lost her battle with breast cancer. Roseanne had always been a very loving, kind, and full-of-life person. She was always ready to tackle anything that came her way. Roseanne was the mother of four young children when she got the dreaded news that she had breast cancer. It was extra difficult for her since her mother and two sisters had succumbed to the disease.

She fought the battle with grace and dignity and a lot of courage. In the end she lost the fight and her four children were left motherless.

In the years since then, breast cancer still has not been cured, although we have come a long way in knowing how to treat cancer successfully. I have family and friends who have had breast cancer and are living healthy and productive lives.

Thank you to the people who work so hard to raise funds and make such a difference to the women who are dealing with this dreadful disease so that they can raise their children and see them become adults, which is every mother's dream.

Toni Slaman

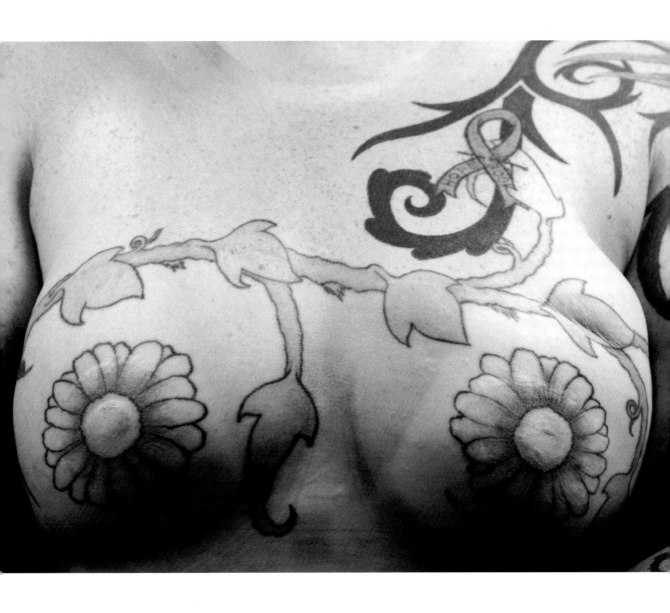

Survivor's Real Bra

I am a young breast cancer survivor, diagnosed at twenty-nine. I had many surgeries (some required, some elective), which ultimately resulted in a double mastectomy followed by implants and chemotherapy. In order to deal with my self-esteem issues, I decided to use creative expression. I sought out a tattoo artist and explained my idea for covering my scars. He said he could do the work and I now have what I show you here. Now I have the confidence to wear low-cut tops and bathing suits. My hope in exhibiting the photo is to give other young women facing breast cancer another option after surgery. Life doesn't end after mastectomy! I am living proof – nine years post treatment, and trying to live life every day to the fullest!

Aimee Horbul

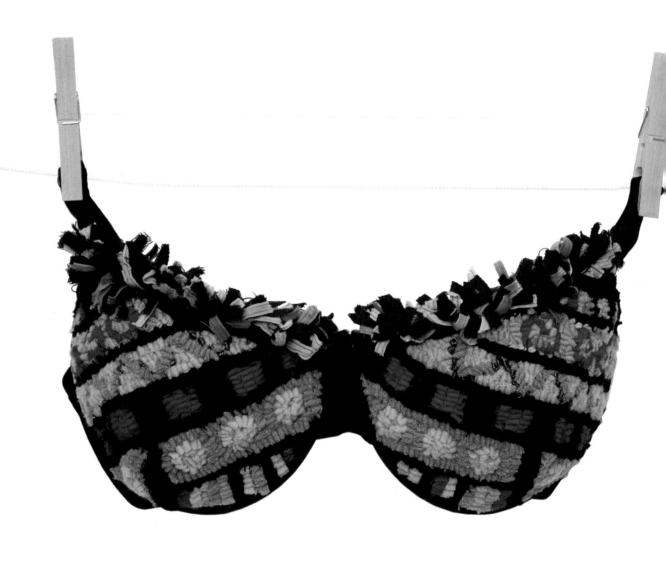

Hooked on Early Screening

When I became aware of this project and saw the Mink and Olympic bras, I knew that I wanted to create a bra in my art form – traditional rug hooking. Using wool strips pulled through a backing with a hook, the same way as rug hookers have done for centuries, I created the cups to attach to a bra. I added bits of glitter and ribbon and an edge done in "proddy," another traditional hooking format. The only tricky part was figuring out how to shape the cups, but I managed to dart and shape them to fit. When I realized that the two cups were not exactly the same, I thought that was okay – no woman has two breasts exactly the same either.

Wendie Scott Davis

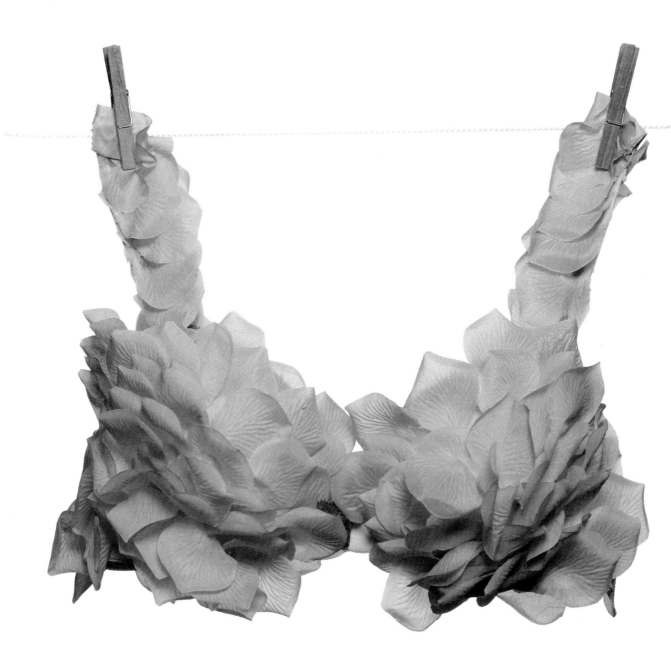

Pink Peddles

I am a six-year cancer survivor. In 2003 I was diagnosed and had a lumpectomy, followed by a round of chemo every twenty-one days for four months and then five weeks of radiation. I developed lymphedema right from the start and still suffer from it today. Now I'm a co-facilitator of our district breast cancer group and a member of a dragon boat team called the Pink Dragons. If there is one thing I've learned, it is that life can be short. Live it to the fullest!

Faye Hanna

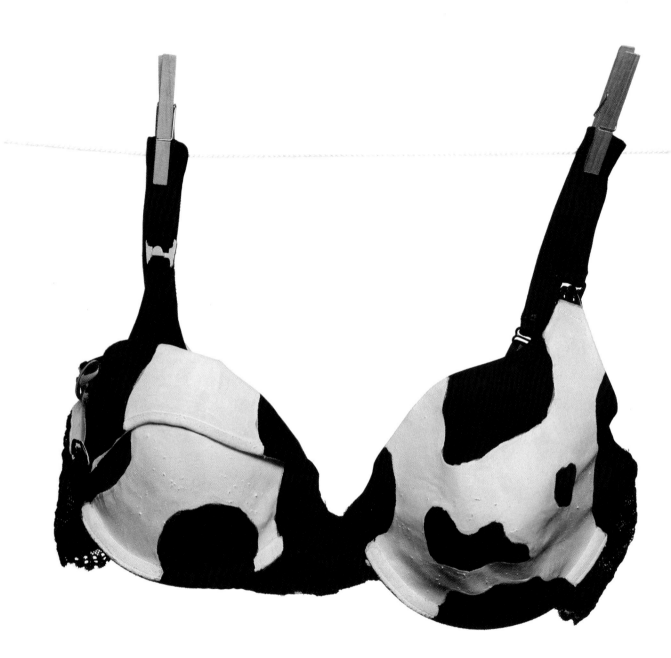

Got Milk?

When I was fifteen years old, I believed my mom would live forever. Then she was diagnosed with breast cancer. She was forty-one. She knew she had a lump in her breast, but the mammogram machine at that time did not detect cancer.

My mom is a fighter, and with the help of many wonderful health-care professionals she was able to beat the cancer. I could have been tested for the two genes that would tell me if I was at a greater risk to develop cancer later in life, but I chose not to know. I do monthly breast self exams, see my doctor yearly, eat well, exercise, and try to maintain a healthy weight – all of which may help decrease my risk of developing breast cancer.

Years later I was at the hospital being told that I was expecting a baby girl. I remember being excited and terrified all at the same time. What if I had passed on the breast cancer gene to my unborn daughter? I began researching about all the wonderful ways breastfeeding can benefit mom and babe – and help reduce the risk of breast cancer.

I now have two girls and a baby boy, resulting in forty months (and counting) of breastfeeding. I believe regular mammography screening on up-to-date equipment will help save my life as well as many other moms, sisters, aunts, grandmas, and best friends. Creating this bra has brought me hope. And, yes, I've got milk!

Carrie Hughes

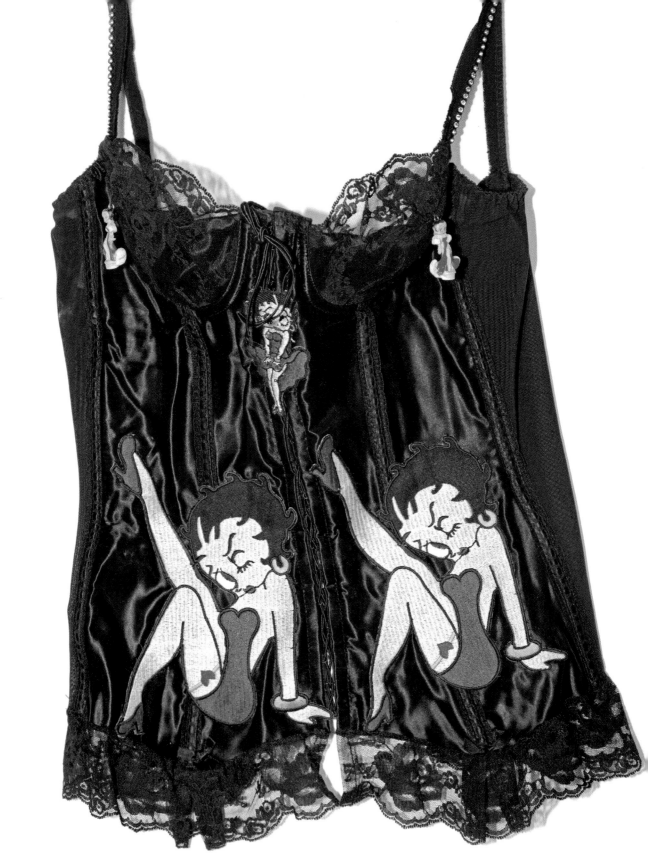

Betty Boobs Booster

Betty Boop has always been a favorite in our family. I have child-hood memories of the comic strips and the occasional Saturday afternoon at the local cinema when a Boop cartoon was shown. When I had my own children, the Saturday morning cartoon shows would sometimes include an old Betty Boop cartoon and both my girls liked Betty. When my eldest daughter was in her teens, she had the Betty Boop shape, including a small "bow" mouth and so we called her Betty Boop and began buying her all manner of Boop memorabilia. Today she has a fair-sized collection. When she saw the "Support the Girls" campaign on the Internet, she told me I should enter. I had an old bustier that had the Boop look, so I decorated it for my daughter and joined the support group.

Mary Lauzon

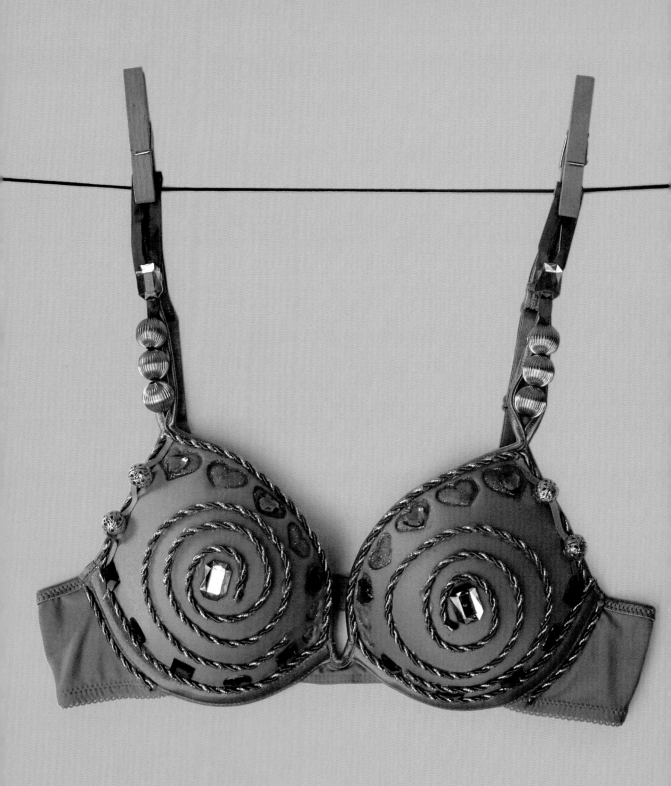

Hidden Treasures

I designed this bra using the colors of royalty and dedicated it to my little princess Meghan, who is one of the treasures in my life. Coming from a family with breast cancer survivors, you learn that life is valuable and should be treasured. Within my family, my great-grandma, two grandmas, and my aunt have all successfully conquered breast cancer. Working as a mammography technologist, I appreciate the importance of such a valuable diagnostic test and have brought this awareness to my mother and my two sisters. One day I will tell my daughter, too. With the advancement in technology, there is hope for early detection and increased survival rates. We need to treasure life because every one of us seems to be impacted by breast cancer somehow, whether it is a family member or a friend.

Hilliary Felsman

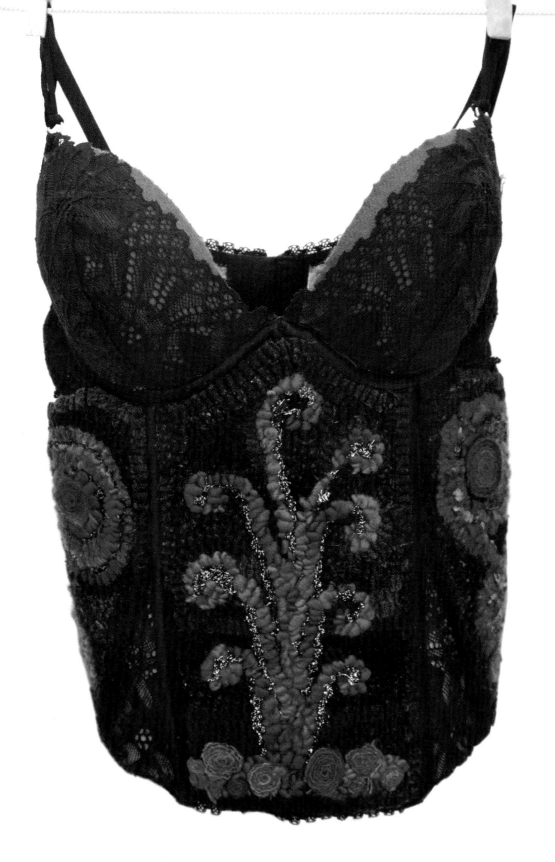

Treading the Maze

I chose a bustier with red accents for this project to acknowledge the innate sexuality of the female breast and the emotional impact of a cancer diagnosis on a woman's psyche.

The side panels represent the spiraling, up, down, in, out – the physical and emotional journey one embarks on when that lump is first suspected. The central panel is a visual reminder of the flames of passion, hope, life, and loving that arise like a phoenix from the ashes of anger, denial, despair, and death.

The flashes of sheen are the "silver linings" behind the clouds, the many unexpected kindnesses from family, friends, and strangers that bolster the spirit and give continued strength to tread the maze of a cancer journey.

This bustier was created to honor friends, both those who survived to wear purple and those who left behind amazing gifts of love, courage, humor, and understanding for their family and friends.

Mary Manuell

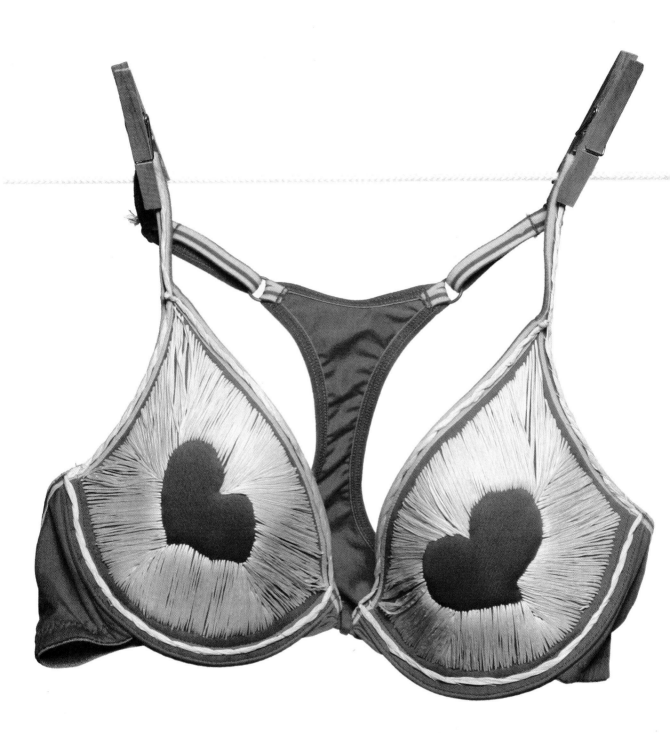

Floss Your Teets

As a dental hygienist, I thought it would be fun to embroider a bra entirely with floss in honor of the patients with cancer (many with breast cancer) I have seen over the years. Good oral health is important during cancer treatment. I educate on the oral implications chemotherapy and radiation can bring about, but my patients teach me so much more. I'm reminded how precious life is and that attitude is everything! I'm dedicating this bra to those patients of mine who didn't win the battle and to those still fighting. Don't forget to 'floss your teets!' (But gently during chemo, please.)

Elaine Dunlop

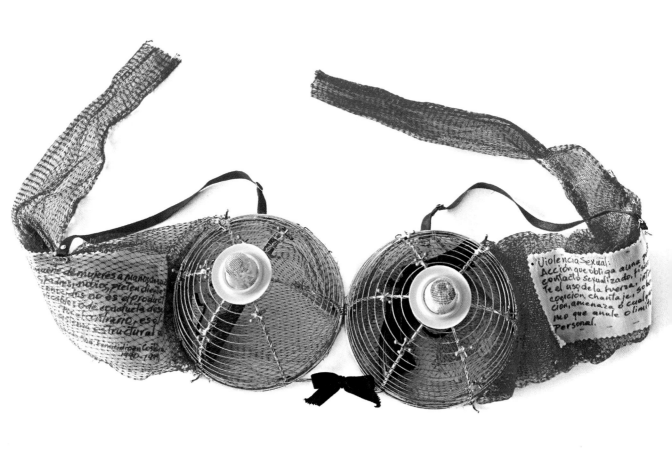

The Tabloid Bra

Tabloid headlines always grab our attention at the supermarket checkout. From celebrity scandals, sex, and violence to the truly bizarre, tabloid newspapers seem to cover stories that are outside the realm of serious journalism.

Tabloids in Costa Rica are filled with sensationalized sexual crimes. Civil society groups have protested, arguing that this portrayal of male-female relations promotes violence against women. That is true, but the law is far from taking any action.

The Tabloid Bra is my representation of this tabloid culture: gun, knife, and kitchen accessories.

Alejandra Gutiérrrez Moya

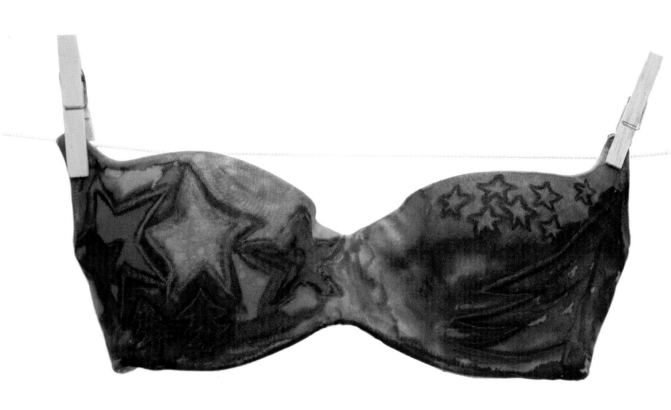

Northern Lights

Nighttime is so magical. I remember being little and wishing upon shooting stars and reading about the mysterious Man in the Moon. I would look up at the night sky on Halloween with visions of witches soaring high, silhouetted against a glowing full moon. On Christmas Eve, I would cross my fingers with hopes of seeing Santa and his reindeer flying through the night on his way to my house.

Our imagination thrives throughout childhood. As we age, we often lose sight of life's magic and, unfortunately, the innocence that makes children embrace such fiction.

Although I'm grown, the night sky will always be full of beauty and intrigue. Having lost my grandma to breast cancer before I was born, I like to envision her at night, when the stars come out. To me, the stars – these bright lights – represent the loved ones we have lost, their presence is forever with us in the magic of the night.

Katie Gibson

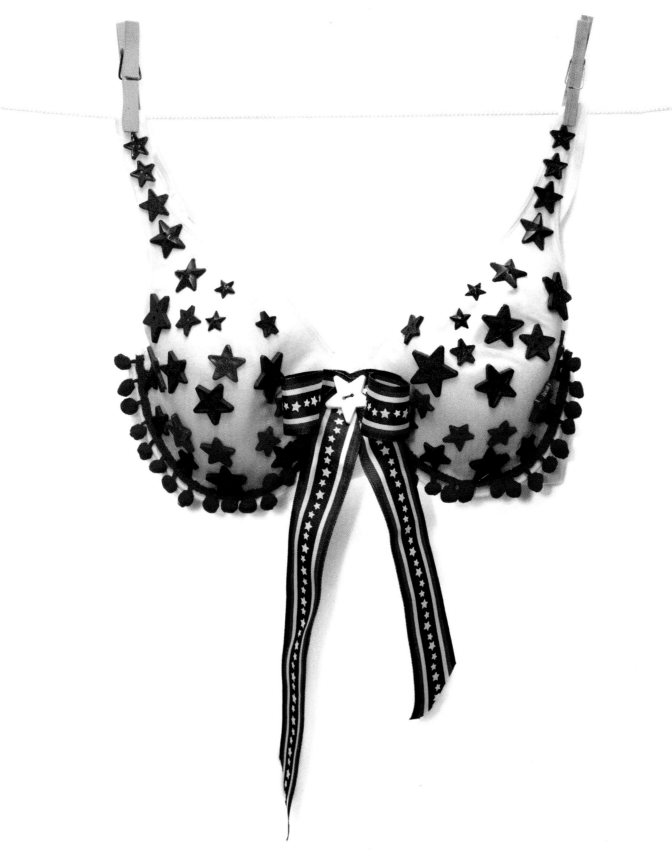

Red, White, and Boobs

My niece, Faye Hanna, is a breast cancer survivor. She visited us here in Florida with her family members last spring. While they were here, each of us made up a bra for them to take back home to Canada. My bra was red, white, and blue for the USA, as many struggle with cancer here. My son's wife is a survivor and is doing well. I pray that one day there will be a cure or quick treatment for all cancers. I had one little scare myself years ago, but thankfully it was only a cyst.

Mary Foster

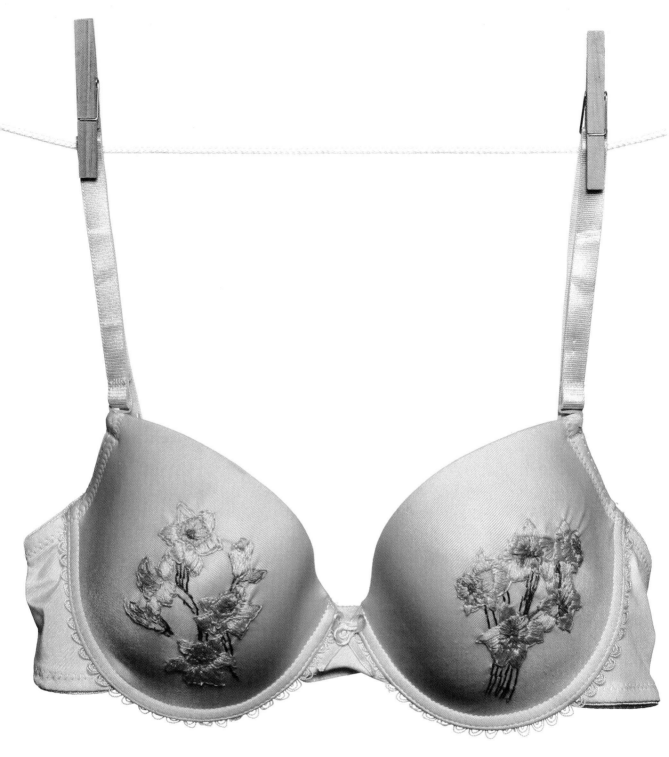

Daffodils

Daffodils have been a symbol for the Canadian Cancer Society since the 1950s when volunteers organizing a fundraising tea decorated the tables with daffodils. The cheerful flowers seemed to radiate hope and faith that cancer could be beaten. Soon the Society realized that the sale of daffodils would generate additional revenue.

Cancer has touched my life too abundantly. In my thirties, my sister-in-law was diagnosed with breast cancer and when she passed away, we took her three teenaged boys into our home.

Since then we have been touched by the cancer of a number of relatives and too many friends. Most recently, our daughter was diagnosed with breast cancer and chose to have a bilateral mastectomy. She stayed at a facility called Daffodil Lodge during her radiation treatments.

When my sister-in-law was diagnosed many years ago, the Canadian Cancer Society symbol was the daffodil and their slogan was "Cancer Can Be Beaten." Today's slogan is "Let's Make Cancer History," but the daffodil still remains to radiate hope and faith that cancer can be beaten.

Carol Ann Nicksy

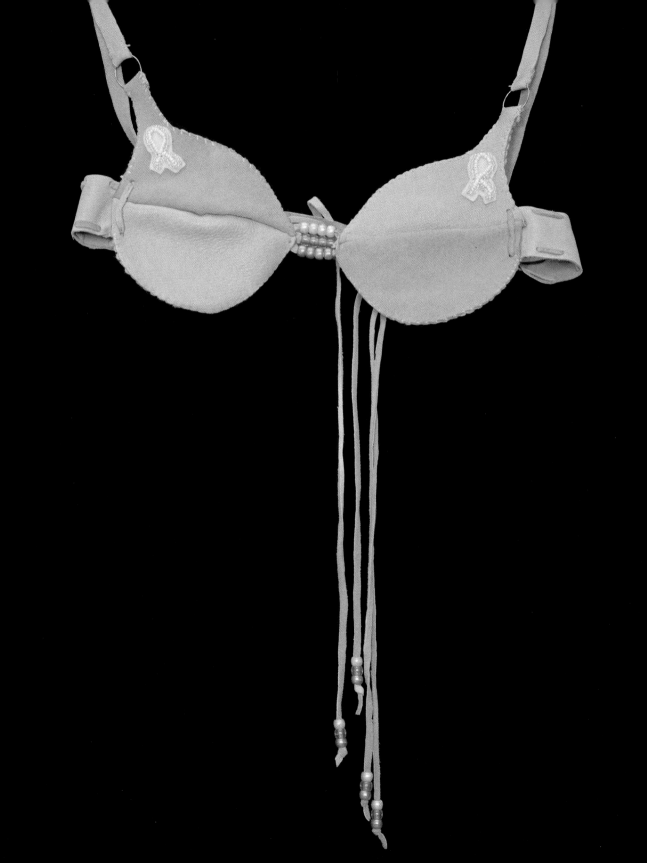

The Friendship Bra

The staff and volunteers at our Aboriginal Friendship Centre sat together and contributed to the making of this bra – hence its name.

Our bra was inspired by the First Nation people, as breast cancer can affect anyone of any nationality. The Friendship Bra is made of leather, which represents bravery, love, honesty, kindness, wisdom, respect, and strength. Bravery for the individual living with cancer, love for the love everyone has for one another, honesty for being truthful, kindness for how everyone should be treated, and strength for families who are dealing with a loved one who is affected by cancer. Leather cannot be torn, so the Friendship Bra will last forever, as will the spirit of the loved one.

As long as we practice the teachings together, we will find a cure for breast cancer.

Friendship Centre

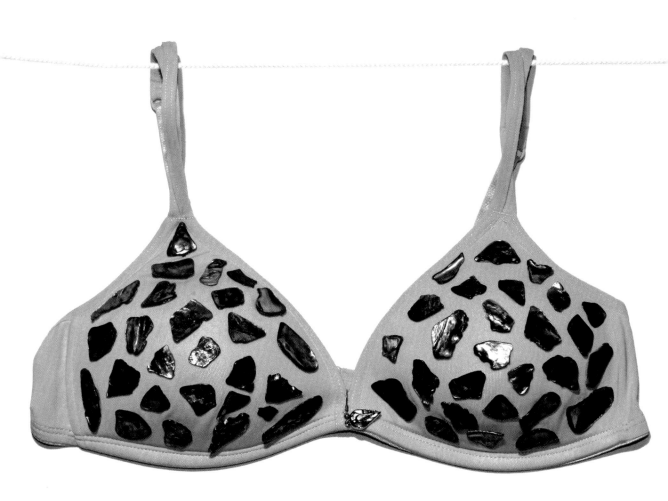

Paua Shells

To celebrate my thirtieth birthday, I booked a bus trip to Europe – solo. I was fortunate to meet many great people but the people I most connected with were from New Zealand.

Fast forward through ten years of keeping in touch and I was headed to New Zealand on vacation. My Kiwi friend drove us from the north of the north island to the south island with an abundance of stops in between.

Paua, which belongs to the same family as abalone, is found exclusively in New Zealand waters and the paua shells are a beautiful reminder of the many hours we spent walking the beaches.

My diagnosis of breast cancer at the age of forty-three was a reminder that life is uncertain and that you should "eat dessert first." Do those things your heart yearns to do before it's too late. Live with no regrets. For me, the paua shell bra represents living life now, not waiting for tomorrow. Isn't it time you went to New Zealand to get your own paua shells, climbed a mountain, spent some time sniffing the roses, or whatever it is that your heart desires?

Karen Campbell

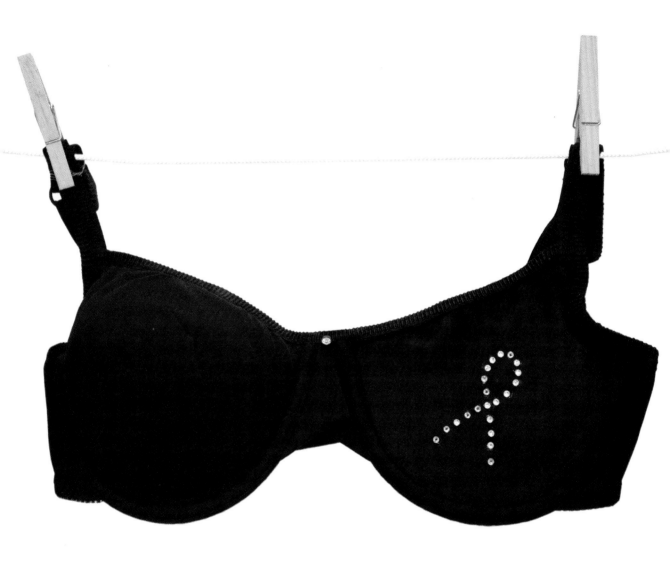

Still Beautiful

I was inspired to contribute to this project after seeing many of the bras hung in the halls of our hospital. There were funny ones, thoughtful ones, and pretty ones, but I did not feel that any spoke to the women who have had a mastectomy. Still Beautiful is a tribute to those women who despite their loss are still mothers, wives, and friends and who can still be complete, sexy, confident women.

Heather Zschogner and the Operating Room Women

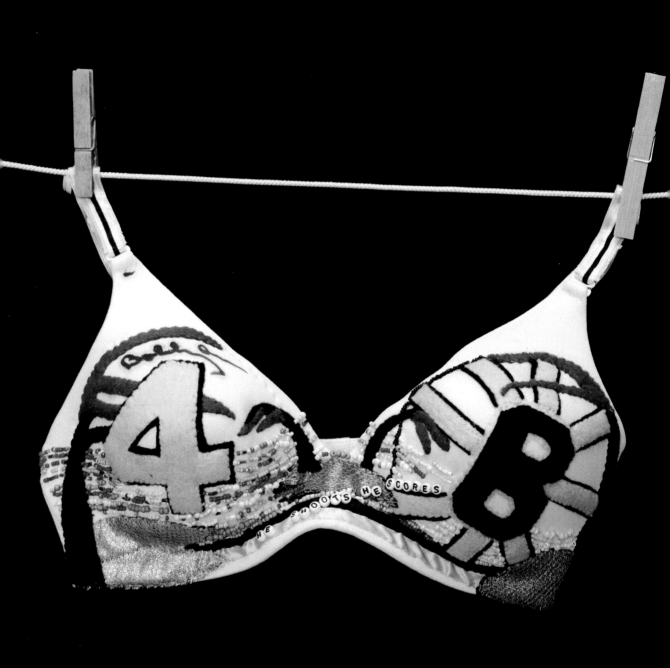

Booby Orr Bra

Cancer touches us all. This bra honors our town's famous son, hockey legend Bobby Orr, and all that our area's geography promises – windswept pines, sparkling blue waters, a lifetime of memories. But perhaps for Parry Sound no memory is greater than May 10th, 1970, when the famous words, "He shoots, he scores!" became etched into our DNA as Bobby's diving goal won the Stanley Cup for the Boston Bruins. Bobby Orr and the Bruins endorsed this bra and they support all that it encompasses. Fighting cancer in remote areas like ours means having the right diagnostic equipment. The bra brings attention to the cause.

Jane Ryder

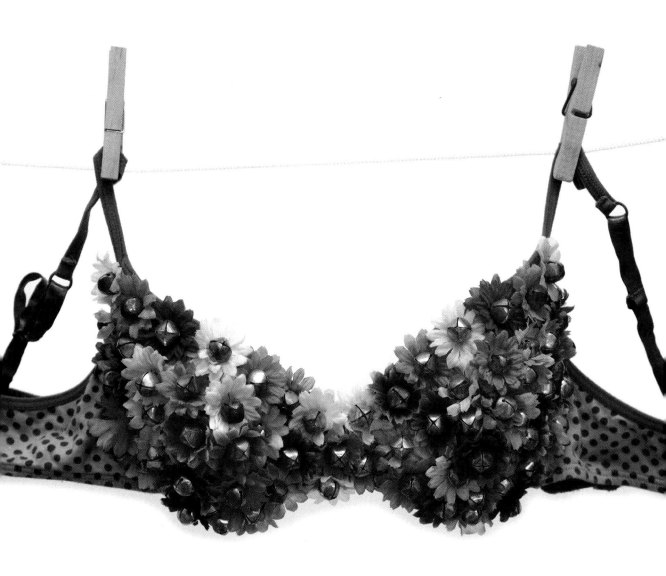

Jingles

Just a few short years ago I met my friend Heather. I had already been very good friends with her sister, Marney, and was caregiver to her mother. The three of us became like sisters. We did many things together – we went on walks together, took trips together, and of course we shopped together, which is where the bells come into the picture. One day while we were in a store, we picked up some colorful bells for some unknown reason and were ringing them in succession creating quite a stir. We had a lot of fun that day. We always laughed when we were together.

In July of 2010, we lost our "Jingles" sister and friend to cancer. Jingles was created in memory of Heather. It reminds me of the laughter and the very good days we had together, rather than the sad times. No matter what came her way, she always looked on the positive side, the funny side.

Carol Ann Cartier

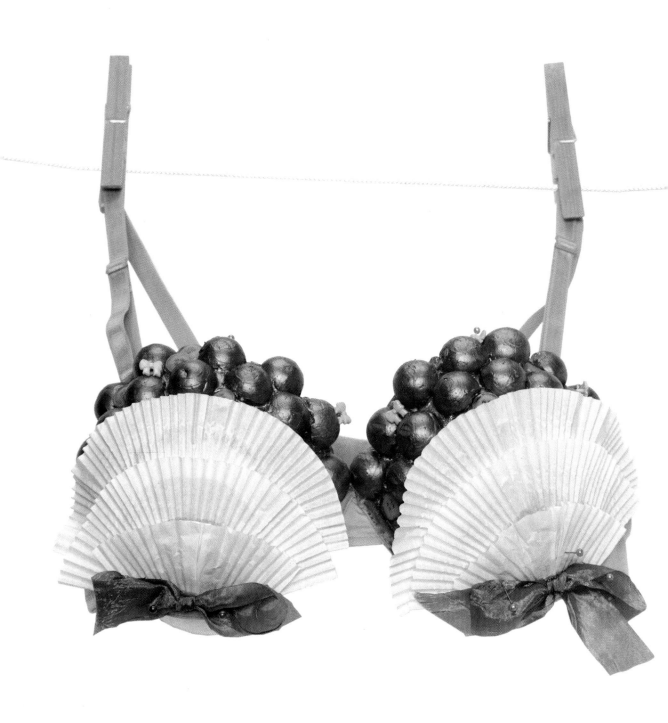

The Cupcake Bra

When I was asked to be the MC for a charity fashion show featuring artistic and whimsical bra designs to raise money for a mammogram machine, I didn't hesitate. I had been designing and producing fashions for forty years and had retired to the community that was embarking on this creative project.

Originally created in 1907, the bra has had my attention throughout my career. In 1964 I actually owned a bra factory and we produced polka dot bras for the Henri Bendel shop in New York City. And in 1967 I had designed a chain bra worn by Samantha Jones on *Sex in the City*.

For the charity fashion show, we decided to start each scene with one of the wonderful bra creations. The bras were our entrance to each fashion scene and they definitely were the stars of the show!

The evening was a great money raiser and the bras were such a hit that I was inspired to design one, too. My latest art show had featured cupcakes – people wearing cupcakes on their heads or carrying them on a tray – so yes, you guessed it. I just had to do the Cupcake Bra.

Marilyn Brooks

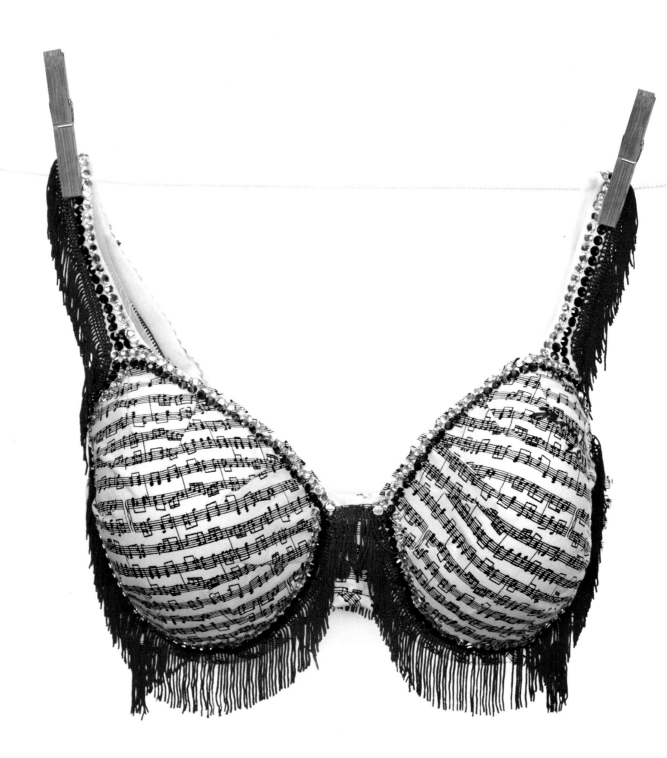

On a High Note

This bra is decorated with music because music was such a big part of the lives of the three very important women in my life who were breast cancer patients.

My best friend Wendy Louza March and I sang together in three quartets as well as in a chorus. Wendy fought a valiant fight against breast cancer for more than a decade, but passed away in 2004.

My sisters, Marney and Sue, and I grew up in a home filled with music. Our grandmother was a singer/actress who supported her children by working, playing the piano at functions, and teaching singing. Every Sunday after dinner she would play the piano and we would sing. Unfortunately, Marney did not get early detection of her breast cancer. She had surgery and extensive chemotherapy, but then had a massive heart attack and passed away.

Daphne Longworth-Smith, my mother, sang with the Sophista-Swings and entertained the troops during WWII. Luckily, I have records of her singing old favorites. Mother had a radical mastectomy in 1992 but was not prescribed chemo or radiation. She survived until 2004.

I am fortunate to have known these three wonderful women. I think about them whenever I hear a song that reminds me of their presence in my life.

Terri Galloway

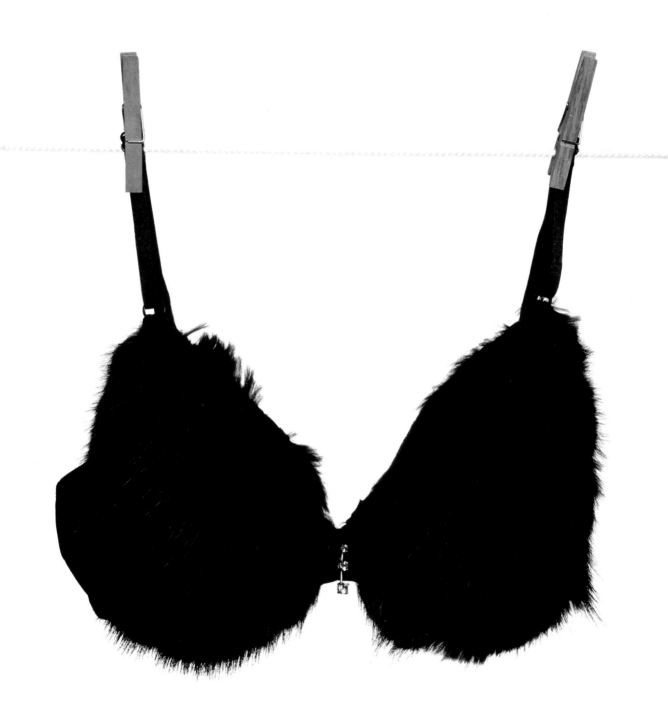

Mink-licious

My inspiration for Mink-licious was our tribe – *us* – women! We support each other, we laugh with each other, we rejoice with each other. We share. We grieve with each other over the loss of one of our tribe taken by breast cancer regardless of her color, creed, nationality, or religion. Even if we didn't know the woman, she was one of us. As a tribe, we can contribute to the early detection and prevention of breast cancer and eventually there will be a cure. Then the rejoicing will be heard around the world.

Susan Tait

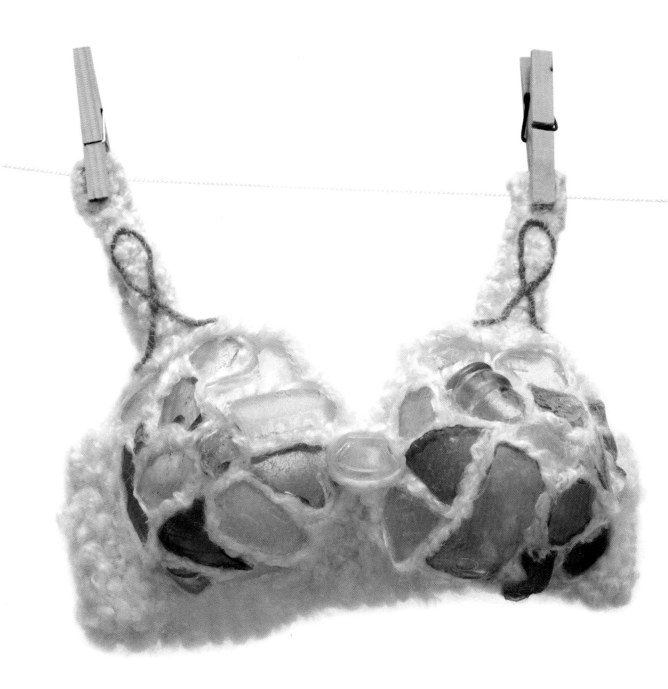

Fragile –
Handle with Care

This bra began as an experiment. I wanted to use a different material to piece my glass creations together, so thought I would try some pink yarn. As I was connecting some pieces, it started to look like a breast, which made me think of the bra project.

I realized that years ago I never knew anyone with cancer and that now I have more friends and relatives touched by this terrible disease than I can mention.

I've had a couple of close calls myself, and I know how it consumes your mind. It's hard to think of anything else, so if having these bras and other pieces of art on display helps distract anyone from their problems, that's a very worthwhile thing to do. I hope my bra can help in some way. I think the name for my creation is very appropriate on many levels.

Debra Strome

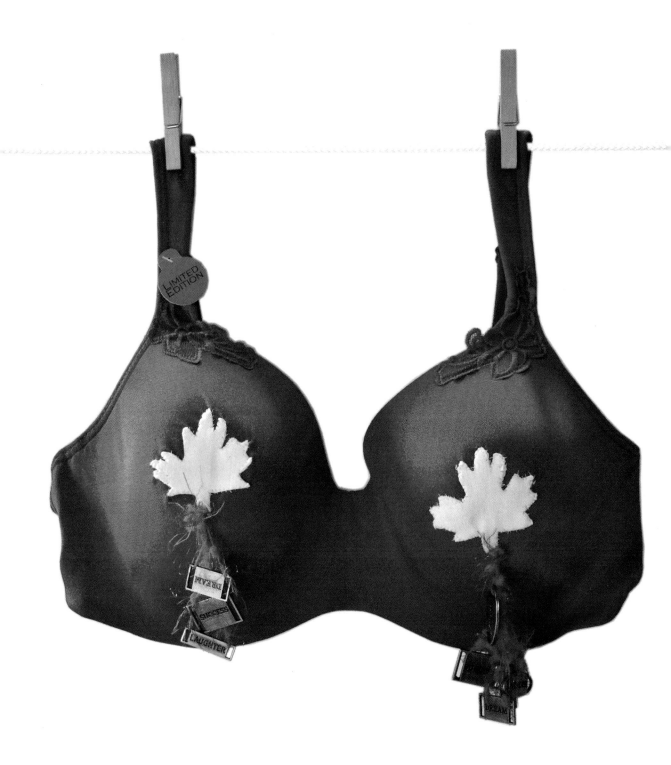

Go Girls, Go!

I had the idea for this bra during the Canada vs US women's hockey game in the 2010 Olympics. Like every other Canadian in February 2010, I was so busy watching the games I could barely get anything else done. Finally, while the rest of the country was watching the men's hockey game, I began to create my art-bra. Making it became a race against time, but I was determined to have it done before the Olympics were over! I missed Sydney Crosby's goal because my head was down sewing the tassels on the maple leaves. (But you can bet I caught the replay!) This bra captures the goodness of the moment – the tassels read 'believe,' 'inspire,' 'wonder.' Terrific words. The bra has caused much delight and laughter in our circles. I never hear the laughs without hearing the lovely character of Lori's voice. There was laughter in her every note. We miss her.

Lynne Atkinson

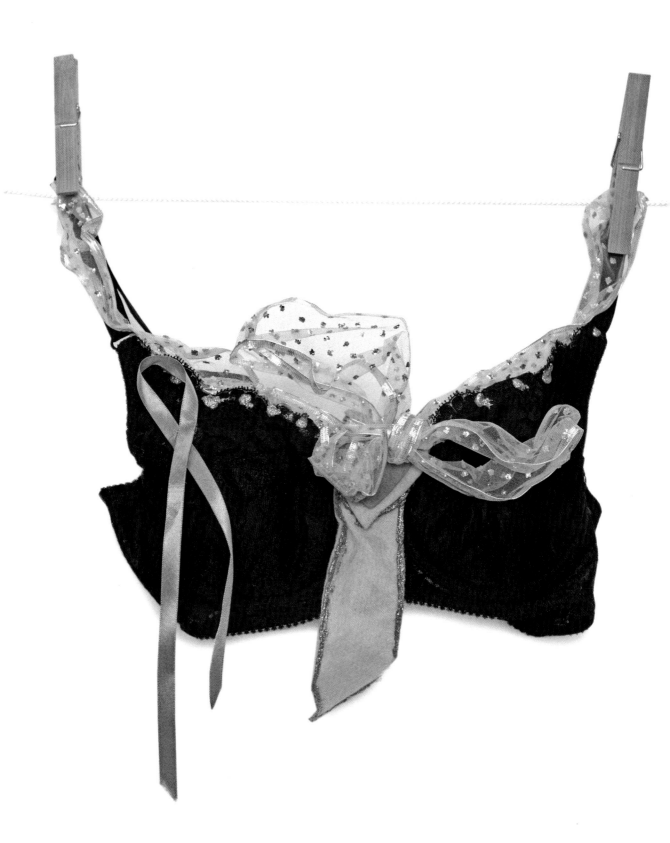

Family Ties

It is very important to know your family history, although for many people this can be a difficult task. There are several types of family history when it comes to breast cancer. If people fall under the hereditary risk pattern, they may be eligible for genetics counseling and then could be tested for specific gene mutations. If anyone – male or female – has inherited a harmful mutation they would be at greater risk of developing different cancers. Routine checkups as well as self-exams could save your life. Know your history, know your body, and stay healthy!

Gail and Bianca Warrilow

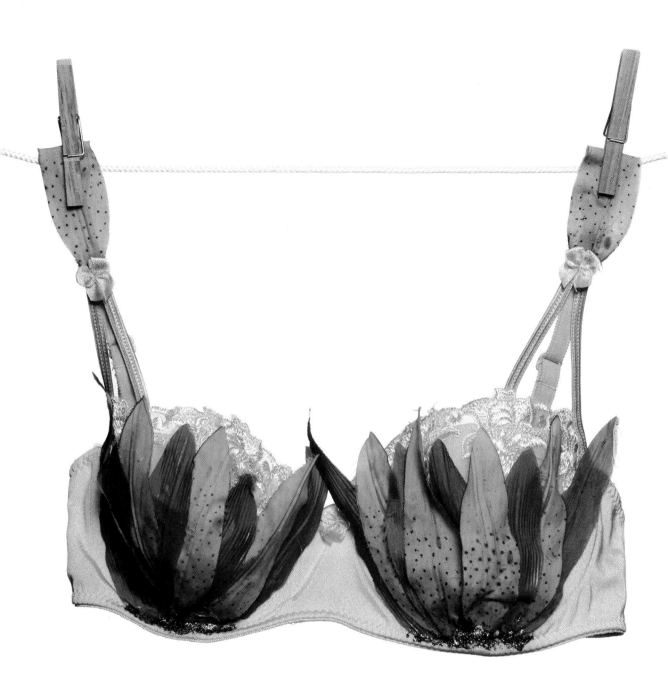

Two Cups of Flower

This bra represents how important it is to follow the recipe to the letter so that the results are excellent. Regular mammograms are the recipe for healthy breasts – and a clean report means so much to each of us. It's like making a cake. If you miss an ingredient, you are taking a big chance on the final results.

We can all become the 'Baker of the Year' by following the instructions given to us by expert medical professionals. Having a mammogram is the most important ingredient; it is the key to early detection and our part in staying cancer free.

Shirley Welling

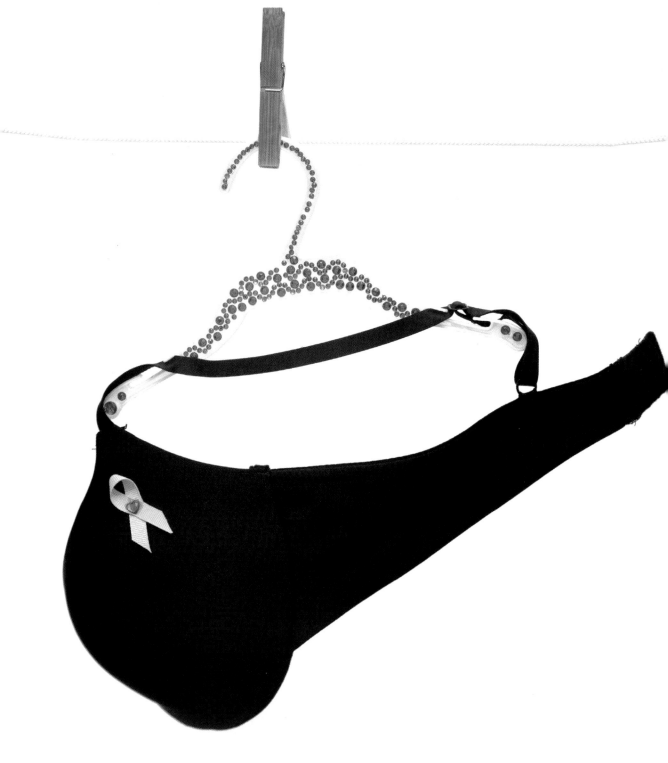

Cups Half FULL

My bra is dedicated to a woman whose name I don't know. I met her in a washroom in a busy bus terminal. At first I didn't pay her much attention; she was busy fussing with herself in front of the mirror. When she asked me for help I saw what she was struggling with – she had lost her hair to chemo and was frantically trying to fix her wig. She wasn't confident that she had reached the perfection she was striving for. I fixed a few of the soft strands that were snagged in the elastic and told her that she looked beautiful. And she did.

To me, this woman is a cup half full. Having obviously overcome a significant battle, there she was in a scruffy bus terminal, breastless and hairless and looking her very best.

This woman is a survivor and to me she represents how far we've come. My bra is not about what is missing but rather what is present. The lady in the washroom seemed to know this. I hope my bra serves as a reminder to seek the full side of the cup in your own life. It's not having two breasts that makes us women, but the inner strength we have within to overcome.

Polly Sutton

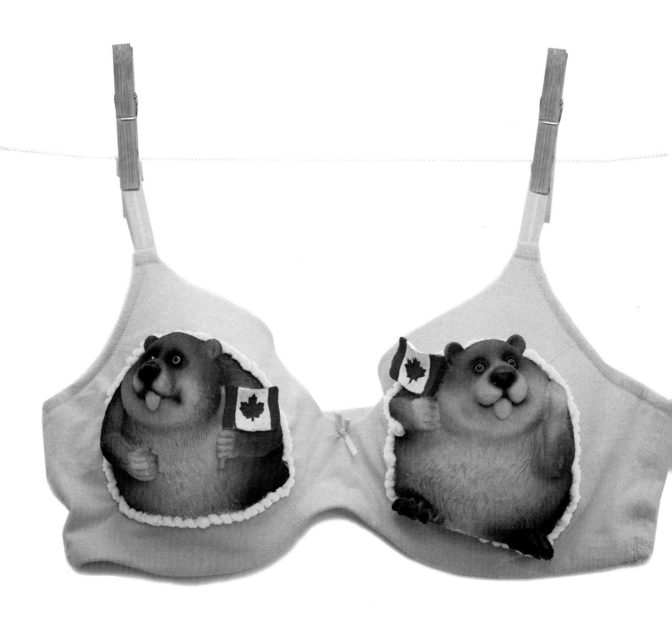

Beaver Boobs

My piece is a tribute to the ethical country we live in and is a playful depiction of the beaver, the symbol we use in Canada to depict our noble, hardworking, and honest nature.

On September 11, 2008, I was diagnosed with a very aggressive form of breast cancer. I can now boast that I am a three-year survivor. One of the wonderful things about Canada is that most of my medical treatments are paid for through our government plan. I did not have to be concerned about where or how to come up with the money to fund my treatments. Yes, I know it comes from paying high taxes but I'll take that any day over greedy insurance companies. The coverage allowed me to concentrate on getting well. Dealing with cancer is a full-time job and no one should have to be concerned as to whether or not they can afford to be sick.

I have heard complaints about our system and the long waits that some have had in receiving medical treatment. I know it has some flaws, but without it I might not be writing about this today. Our healthcare system saved my life.

Josephine Hazen

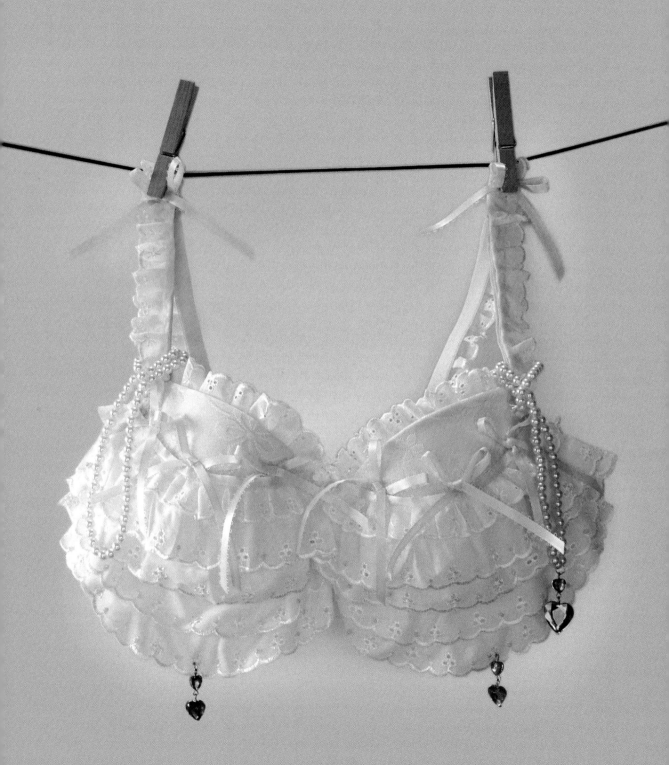

Victory'an Secrets

How should I decorate my bra? What should I call it?

Since I am one of the mammographers at the center that needed the mammography equipment, I really wanted to participate in this event and I wanted my bra to represent something positive.

Finally it came to me – a bra decorated with lace would be very pretty and I could call it "Victorian." The root word of Victorian is "victory" – victory for our more "secret" anatomy over our rival, breast cancer.

It seemed right. Hence Victory' an Secrets.

Marie Shurr

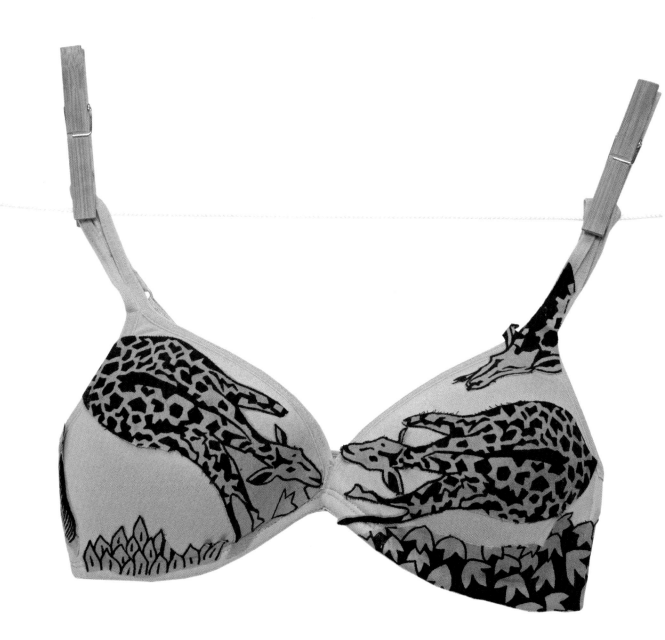

Big Game Hunters

I created this bra in honor of my mother – a breast cancer survivor who succumbed to ovarian cancer. When my lot was to follow in those tracks I went on the big hunt for a course of treatment that would help me win the game and return to good health.

Kathy Krug

Postscript
For two years Kathy led a full life, traveling with husband Ted to the far reaches of the world and participating in the tapestry of offerings her community served up. Throughout this time Kathy had the energy to maintain her vigorous pace with the grace and aplomb that we so loved. She was a beacon in our world. Her light went out October 2011. We miss her.

Lynne Atkinson,
Executive Director,
West Parry Sound Health
Centre Foundation

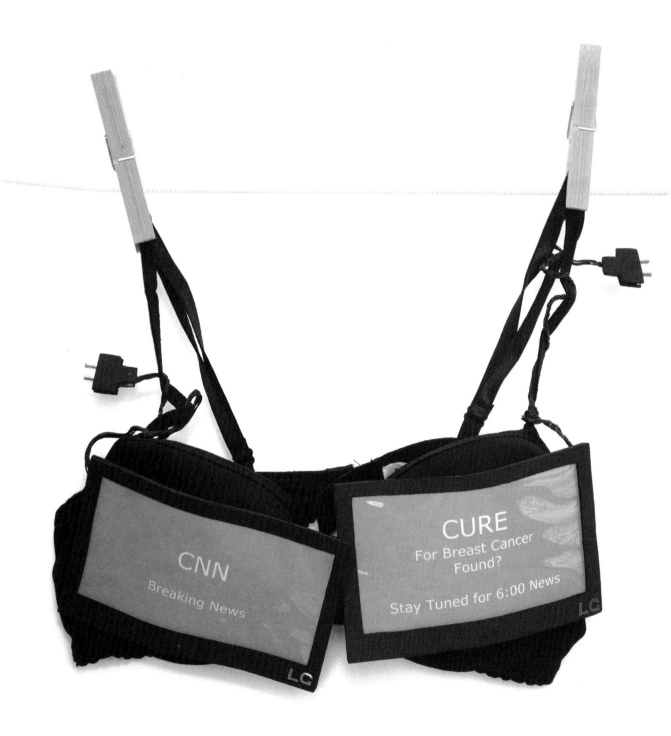

Boob Tube

I found out about this project from my employer, Dr. Corrine Gehrels, a breast cancer survivor and the woman to whom I dedicate the Boob Tube. As well as being an inspiration to all, Dr. Gehrels is also co-chair of the Art-Bra Project. Her enthusiasm and dedication to this fundraiser gave me the incentive to design and submit a bra in her honor. She is truly a very courageous and remarkable person.

Boob, a.k.a. breast, and the Tube, a.k.a. television, seem to have one thing in common – they both get lots of attention and ATTENTION is what is needed to broadcast the message that awareness and continued fundraising for breast cancer is so important and so vital to the cause.

Annette Turriff

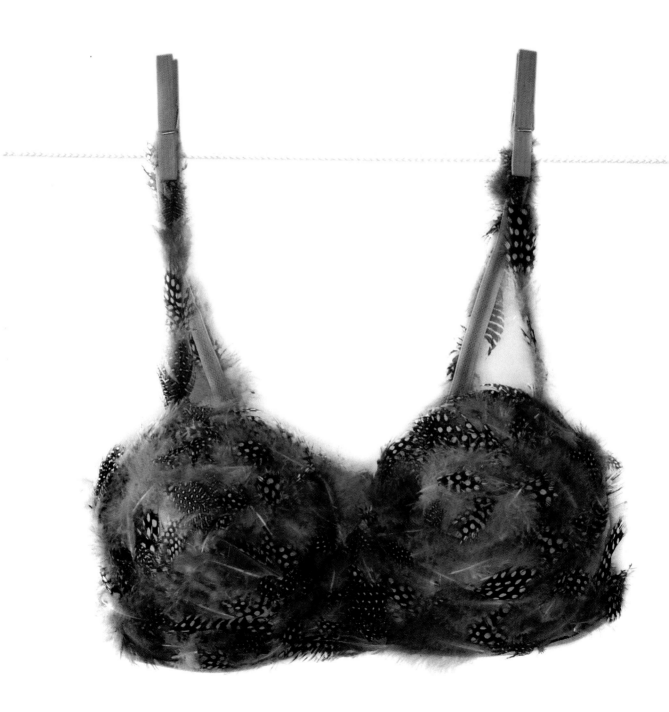

Birds of a Feather

As a co-facilitator of our local Breast Cancer Support Group I feel this bra represents all women who have undergone breast cancer. We all get together to help each other stay strong and positive throughout our recovery.

We learn from each of these women when they share the experiences they have gone through. Telling their stories helps them as well as the rest of us.

Like the feathers of a bird we are very dependent on each other. We do not want to lose even one feather.

Shirley Welling

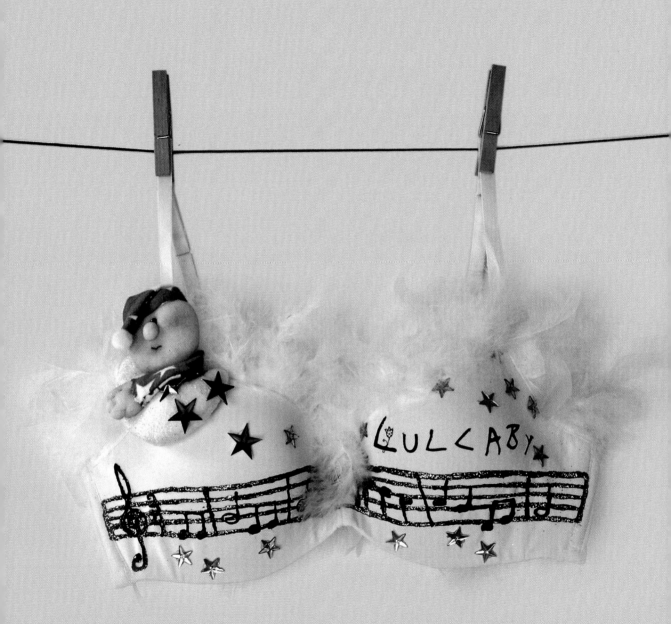

BRAhms Lullaby

After watching my sister go though treatment at the age of forty-two, and knowing that my aunt had died of breast cancer at the age of thirty, I decided to have genetic testing. I learned that I have a mutation that gave me a fifty to eighty-five percent chance of getting breast cancer.

The community at www.facingourrisk.org helped me to weigh my options and connect with other women who are at high risk of breast cancer. After much research and consideration, I decided to have preventative surgery, and was able to reduce my risk of breast cancer to less than two percent. I am deeply grateful that I was able to learn about my cancer risk and act on that knowledge to protect my health. Knowing that I have reduced my risk so significantly has brought me such great peace of mind!

BRAhms lullaby – a familiar tune – is accompanied by wishes of rest and peace for you, wherever you are in your journey.

Betty Ann Reid, with Emma and Erin Reid

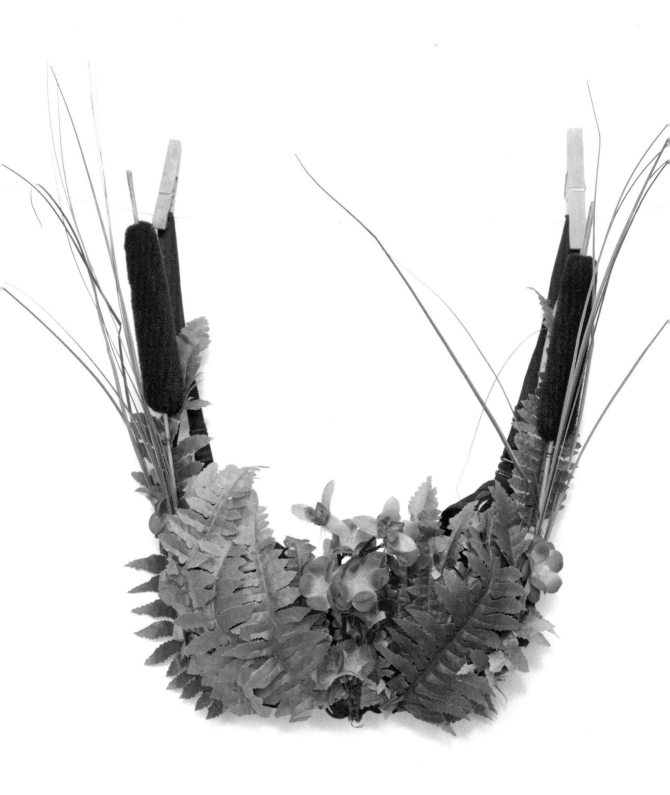

Antheia

My daughter Shelby and I decided to help show our support for fundraising to buy a digital mammography machine by designing bras for the project.

We wanted to help spread the message that we are all connected through our need to support "The Girls." We named our creation for the Greek goddess Antheia because she was the goddess of vegetation, marshlands, gardens, blossoms, the budding earth, and human love. We chose this theme because we are inspired by nature and the infinite healing capabilities that nature offers.

Karen Mahon

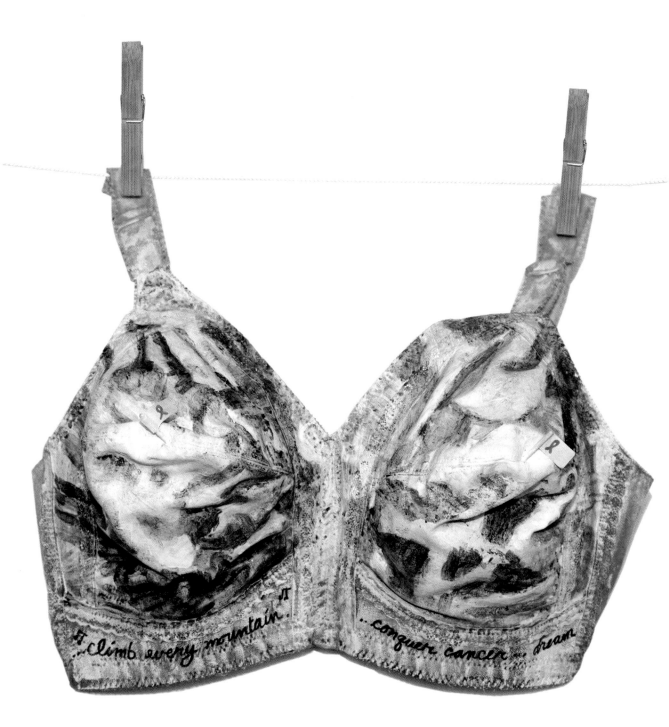

Climb Every Mountain, Conquer Cancer Dream

When I heard about this project, I quickly visualized an art piece. Finding a suitable bra was fun – I searched out a super stiff, pointed, large-cupped specimen to be a good base for my vision.

The symbolic parallel of climbing a mountain and placing a flag with the breast cancer logo on it seemed fitting. The character required of someone who takes on a challenge to conquer, whether it be climbing a mountain or facing a cancer, is admirable. Taking on the task with dignity, strength, and courage and overcoming obstacles with determination and focus is the inspiration for this piece.

The title is inspired by the song from the movie *The Sound of Music*, with its message to face challenges, fears, and insecurities head on "…till you find your dream." A perfect theme song for our dream of conquering cancer.

Jane Jones

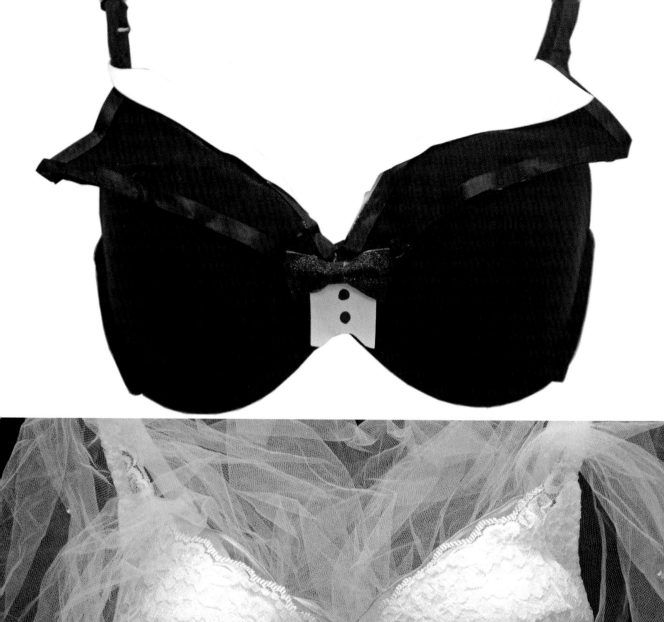

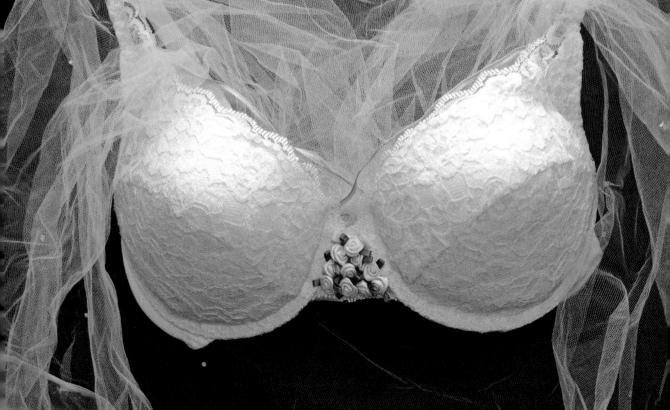

A Black Tie Affair

As an event planning business, we at A Black Tie Affair were inspired to create awareness for this project by hosting the first ever Brides' Ball in our community. The idea of the ball was to encourage women to pull out their wedding gowns or bridesmaid dresses and for men to suit up for an evening of entertainment, community spirit, and glamour. The bride and groom bras symbolize the fact that both men and women are affected emotionally and physically by breast cancer. This project truly reflects the power of numbers. It started in a small community and has created awareness worldwide. It has been an honor to be a part of it.

Tanis Mack and Amy Black

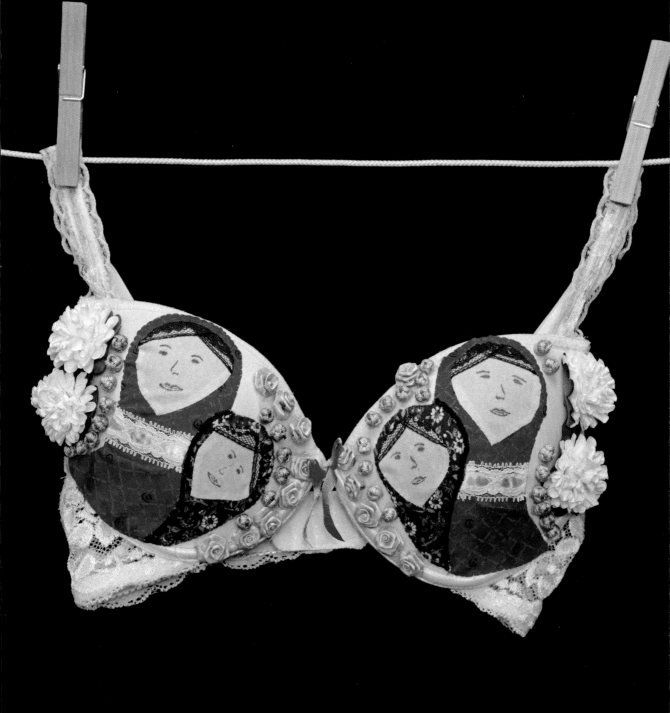

Girls in the Garden

This bra was made in memory of my sister-in-law who died of breast cancer in 1966. She was disabled after contracting polio when she was very young and lived with us until her death.

At the time, we lived in a place with a very secluded yard that had mature trees and a rock garden and it was always her delight when she could gather all the girls in the family to sit in the garden with her to enjoy the sunshine and the surroundings.

Liz Hugli

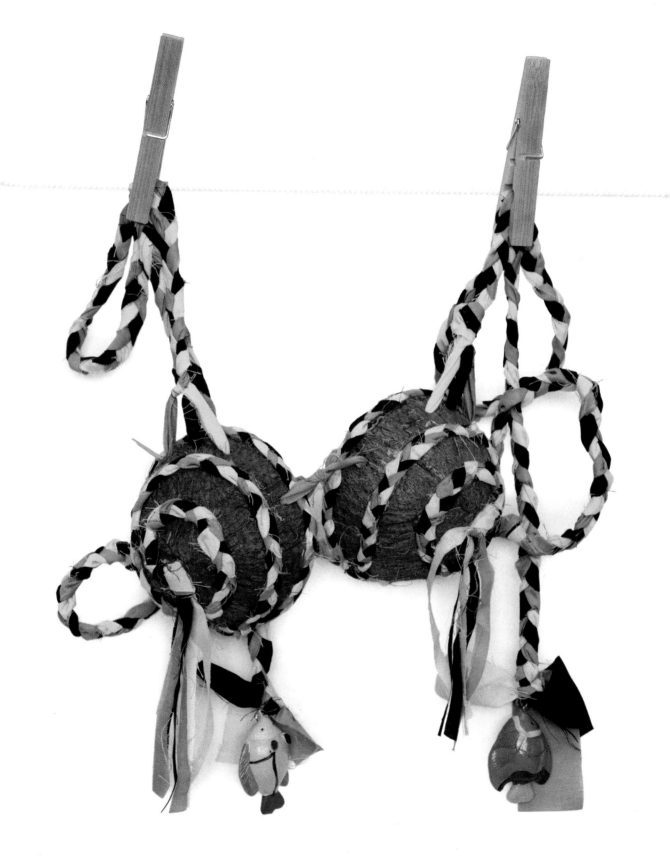

BRAhama Mama

I was born in the Bahamas and my mother is a breast cancer survivor. The Bahamas is a small country with a population of only 338,000. It is purported to have an unusually high incidence of breast cancer among its young women. Recent studies have indicated that there is a genetic connection to this finding.

I made this bra using the colors of the Bahamian flag to represent the Bahamian women, the coconuts to represent their sense of humor and vibrant personalities, and the umbrellas to protect them from the occurrence of this disease.

Christina Cox

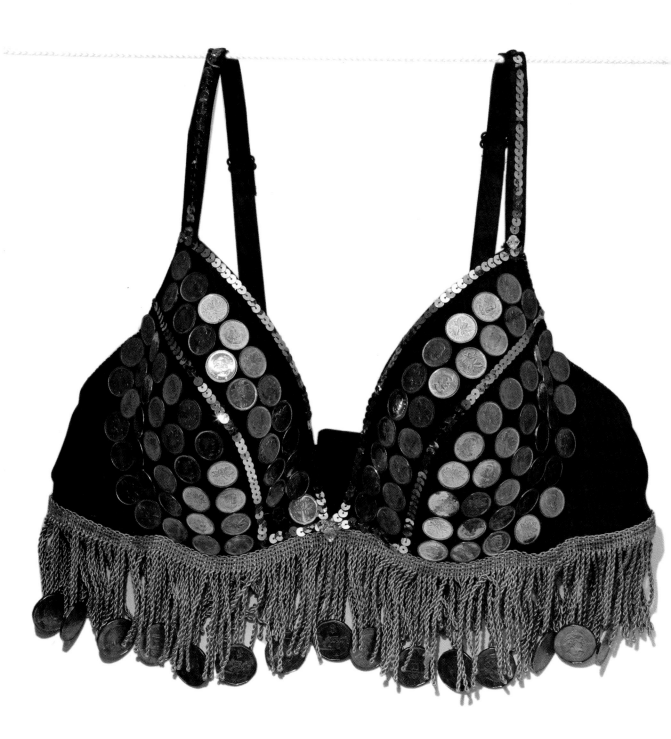

Cha-Ching

The staff of our credit union was inspired to make this art-bra for several reasons. We have loyally participated in various fundraising efforts over the years and this project involved no paddling or running so it was an instant hit! Only our creativity was challenged. We went with the obvious theme for a financial institution – money! We hoped the eye-catching bra would help raise awareness of the campaign and bring in the funds to buy the much needed digital mammography equipment.

Cancer has touched our work family and, consistent with our culture, our branch has always rallied around the affected staff member by holding fundraisers or contributing to them. Not all these stories had happy endings. The art-bra initiative represents hope that with new technology, there will be more successes to celebrate.

Last but not least, all our staff members are female so the importance of early detection of breast cancer is not lost on us. We hope our bra also leaves you with the overriding impression that it makes "cents" to have a mammogram!

Debbie, Lorraine, Brenda, Rachel,
Sandra, Christie-Lynn, Lina, Tiffany, April
The Women from the Kawartha Credit Union

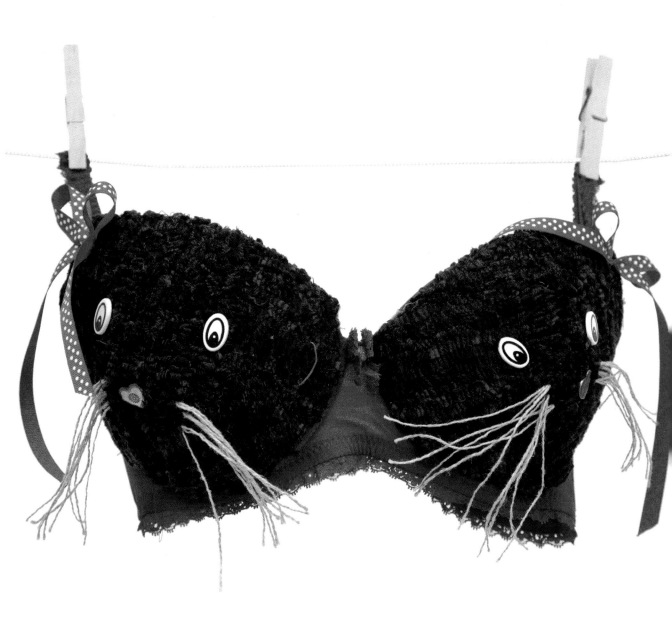

Plaid Pals

This bra is named Plaid Pals because it represents the friendship between women. The plaid was given to me by a special friend when I was looking for old woolen clothes to cut up for my hooking projects. During times of cancer, the friendship between women helps them become stronger. "Pal" also refers to our pets (this one being a cat) who hold a special place in our healing journeys. This bra is dedicated to my friends Doreen, who has been cancer free for more than ten years, and Marj, who is receiving chemo right now. Together we can make a difference!

Barbara Vaughan

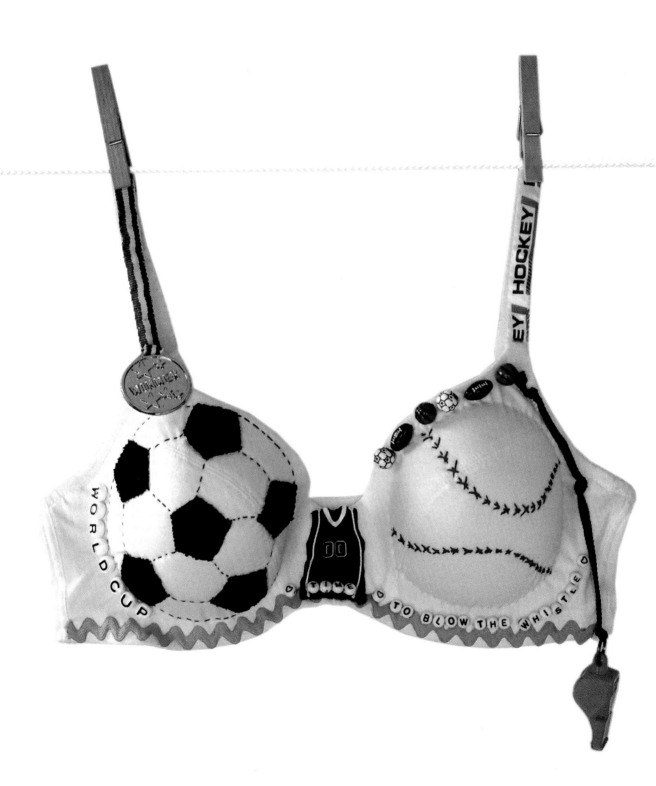

Sports Bra

Inspired by the good friends I have known who have courageously fought the cancer battle, and in memory and honor of my dear mother-in-law, Lois Ryder, I designed a bra to celebrate the team effort we need to raise awareness and support for all types of cancer – but in particular breast cancer.

My message is this: It's time to blow the whistle on cancer! Working as a team we can make a difference. We need to make our goal early screening and detection, so that treatment can begin as soon as possible. Even though cancer is a disease that doesn't seem to play by the rules, with tenacious team spirit, we can be victorious!

Jane Ryder

Acknowledgments

The art-bras you see in this book were crafted to bring solace and yes, even laughter to the viewer. On March 6, 2010, the first two art-bras were modeled at a Georgian Bay International Women's Day event. Just over a year later, 101 of the whimsical creations, with their accompanying stories, were installed on the walls throughout our small-town hospital two-and-a half hours north of Toronto, Ontario. The installation became the eye candy for our successful digital mammography fundraising campaign. The journey from idea to execution was a great ride and offered much to be thankful for along the way.

I wish to express deep appreciation to Susan Tait (Manager of the Georgian Bay Women's Network), Paula Attwell (campaign co-chair) and Dr. Corrine Gehrels (campaign co-chair). All three of these women propelled our campaign into the stratosphere with their expertise, faith, and doggedness in getting the job done. A special thanks to Zis Parras. Because of Zis, our Support the Girls project was invited to the 2011 Canadian National Exhibition in Toronto, where thousands saw and reacted to our art-bras. This would not have happened without the generous support of the Parry Sound Community Business and Development Centre, which made it financially viable for us to travel our art installation physically and virtually. Thank you. And thanks to the West Parry Sound Health Centre CEO, Donald Sanderson, for saying 'Yes' to the kooky idea of hanging art-bras on clotheslines around our hospital. A very special thanks must go to the many bra-artistas who filled those lines and shared their stories and to our five photographers, three local, one from Winnipeg, and one from Costa Rica, whose photos have memorialized the art-bras: Ted Krug, Delia Brereton, Cody Storm-Cooper, Darcy Finely, and Marcela Valdeavellano. Finally, I want to thank our publisher Margie Wolfe and Second Story Press for their belief that our community art project installed in a small town in Northern Ontario had something to share with people around the world.

Lynne Atkinson
Executive Director,
West Parry Sound Health
Centre Foundation

Photo Credits

Mums Forever: Cody Storm Cooper
Fly High: Cody Storm Cooper
Stone Age Bra: Ted Krug
Cradles Of Civilization: Cody Storm Cooper
Hole in One: Ted Krug
Training Bra: Ted Krug
Savvy 'DDD' Lite: Ted Krug
Lucky Charms: Cody Storm Cooper
Friends Forever: Ted Krug
Survivor's Real Bra: Darcy Finley
Hooked On Early Screening: Ted Krug
Pink Peddles: Cody Storm Cooper
Got Milk?: Cody Storm Cooper
Betty Boobs Boostier: Ted Krug
Hidden Treasures: Delia Brereton
Treading the Maze: Ted Krug
Floss Your Teets: Cody Storm Cooper
The Tabloid Bra: Marcela Valdeavellano
Northern Lights: Ted Krug
Red, White, And Boobs: Ted Krug
Daffodils: Cody Storm Cooper
The Friendship Bra: Ted Krug
Paua Shells: Cody Storm Cooper

Still Beautiful: Ted Krug
Booby Orr Bra: Ted Krug
Jingles: Ted Krug
The Cupcake Art Bra: Ted Krug
On a High Note: Ted Krug
Mink-licious: Cody Storm Cooper
Fragile - Handle With Care: Ted Krug
Go Girls, Go!: Delia Brereton
Family Ties: Ted Krug
Two Cups of Flower: Cody Storm Cooper
Cups Half FULL: Ted Krug
Beaver Boobs: Ted Krug
Victory'an Secrets: Delia Brereton
Big Game Hunters: Ted Krug
Boob Tube: Ted Krug
Birds of a Feather: Delia Brereton
BRAhms Lullaby: Delia Brereton
Antheia: Ted Krug
Climb Every Mountain Conquer Cancer Dream: Ted Krug
A Black Tie Affair: Ted Krug
Girls In The Garden: Ted Krug
BRAhama Mama: Ted Krug
Cha-Ching: Cody Storm Cooper
Plaid Pals: Ted Krug
Sports Bra: Delia Brereton